The Little Girl Who Loved Sweets

FOR LITTLE CHILDREN

WHO WISH TO HAVE

HAPPY TEETH

AND

A PRETTY SMILE.

Once upon a time there was a
little girl.......

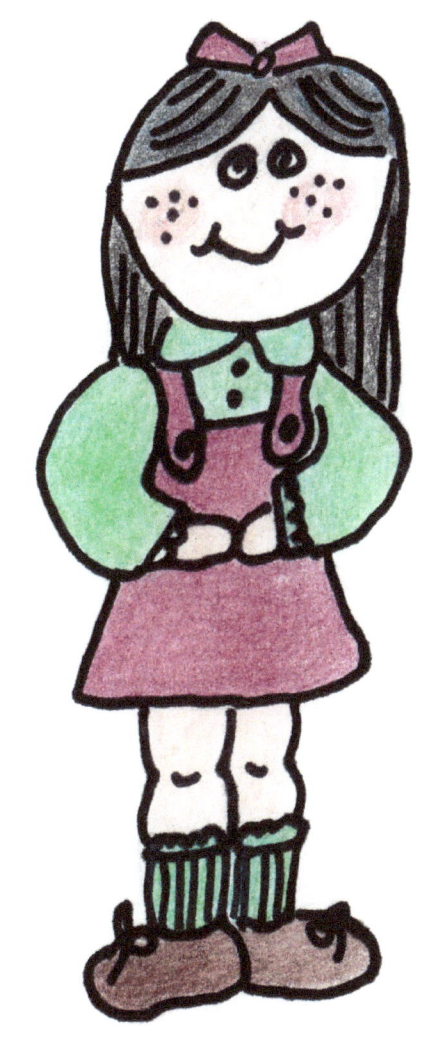

Who loved sweets.

She ate sugar coated cereals, doughnuts, or waffles dripping in sweet syrup for breakfast.

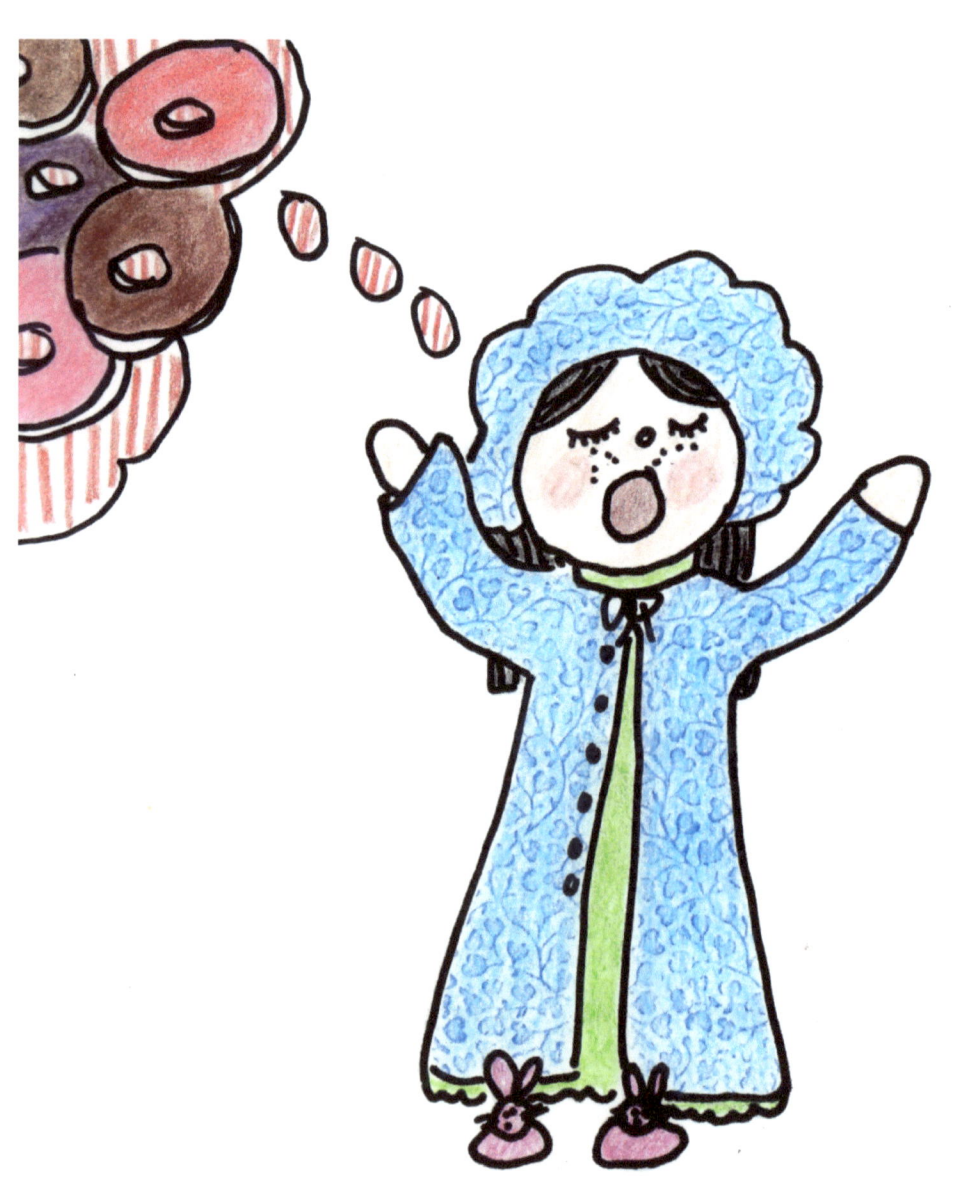

She snacked on candy all afternoon.

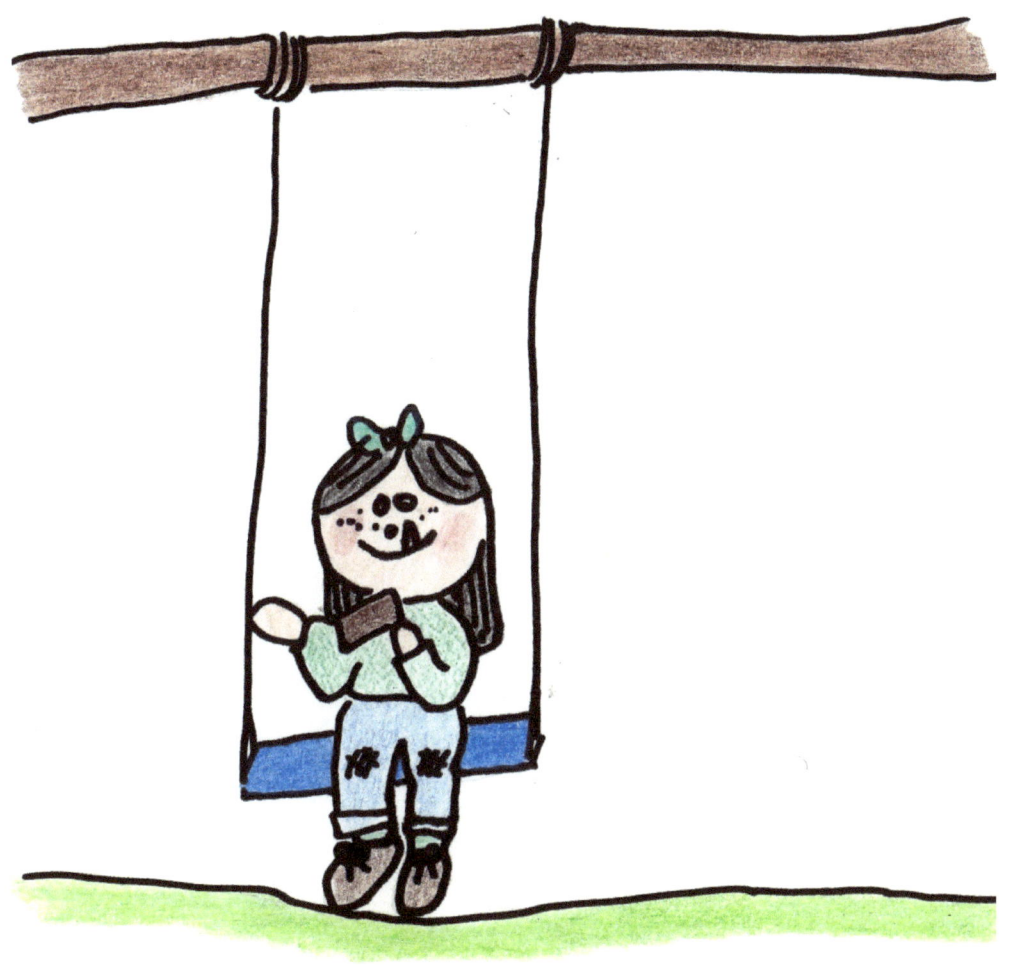

She chewed chewing gum while watching TV.

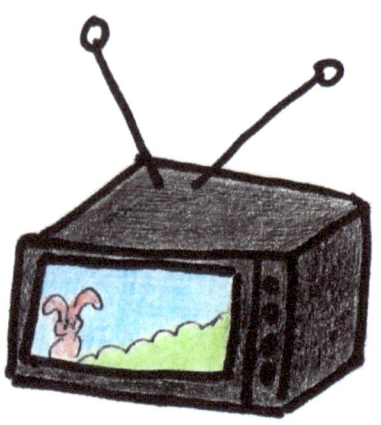

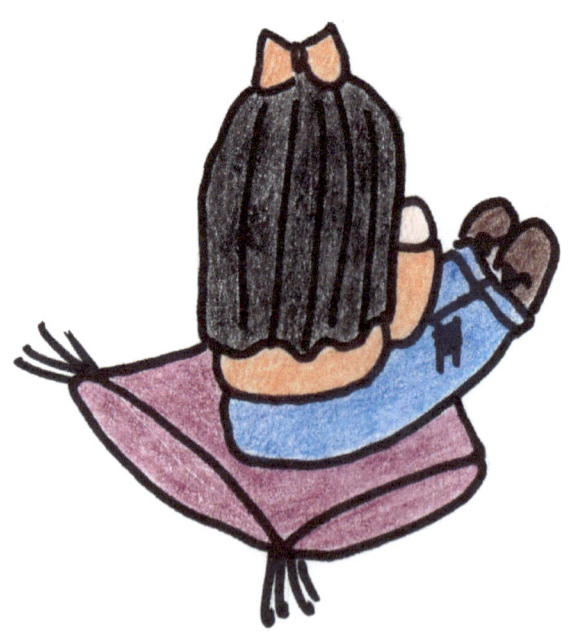

She ate cookies with her milk
before she went to bed.

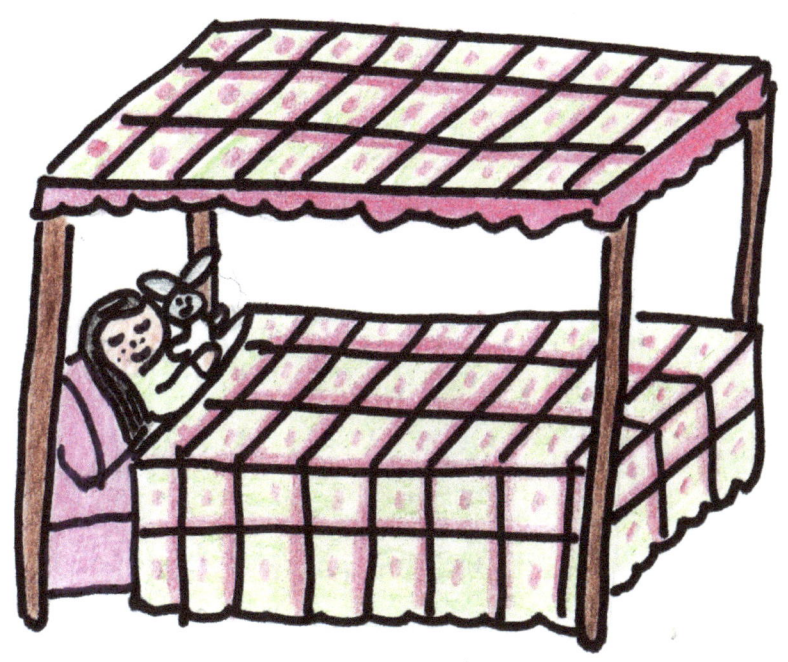

One day she heard a tiny voice
calling her name from
inside her mouth.

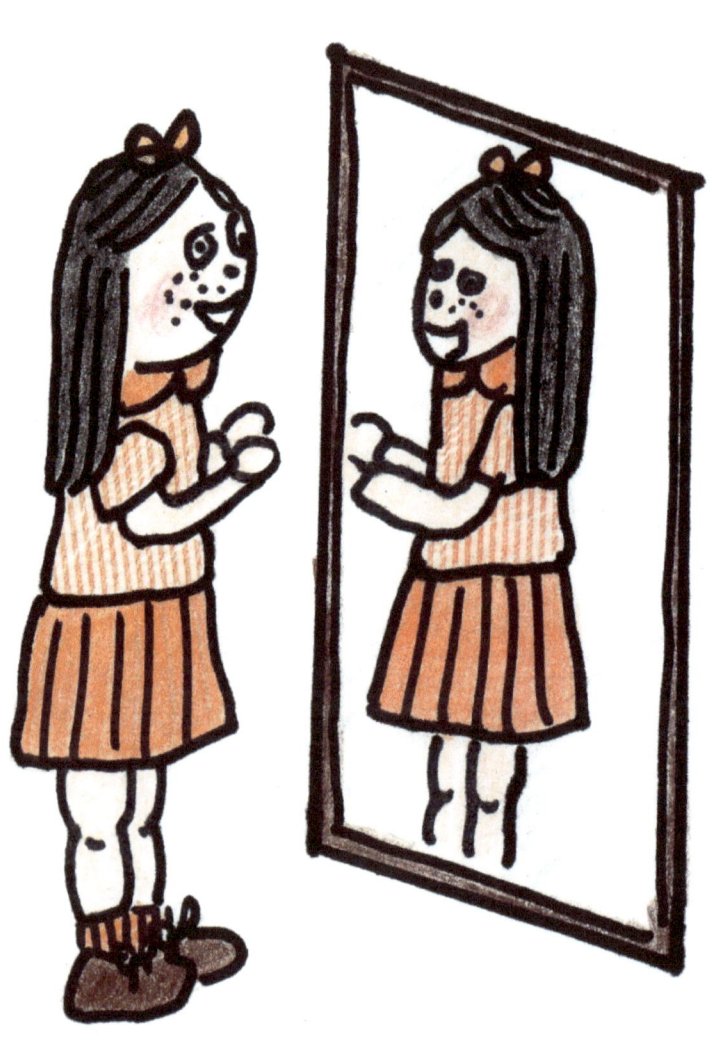

She ran to the mirror and looked.

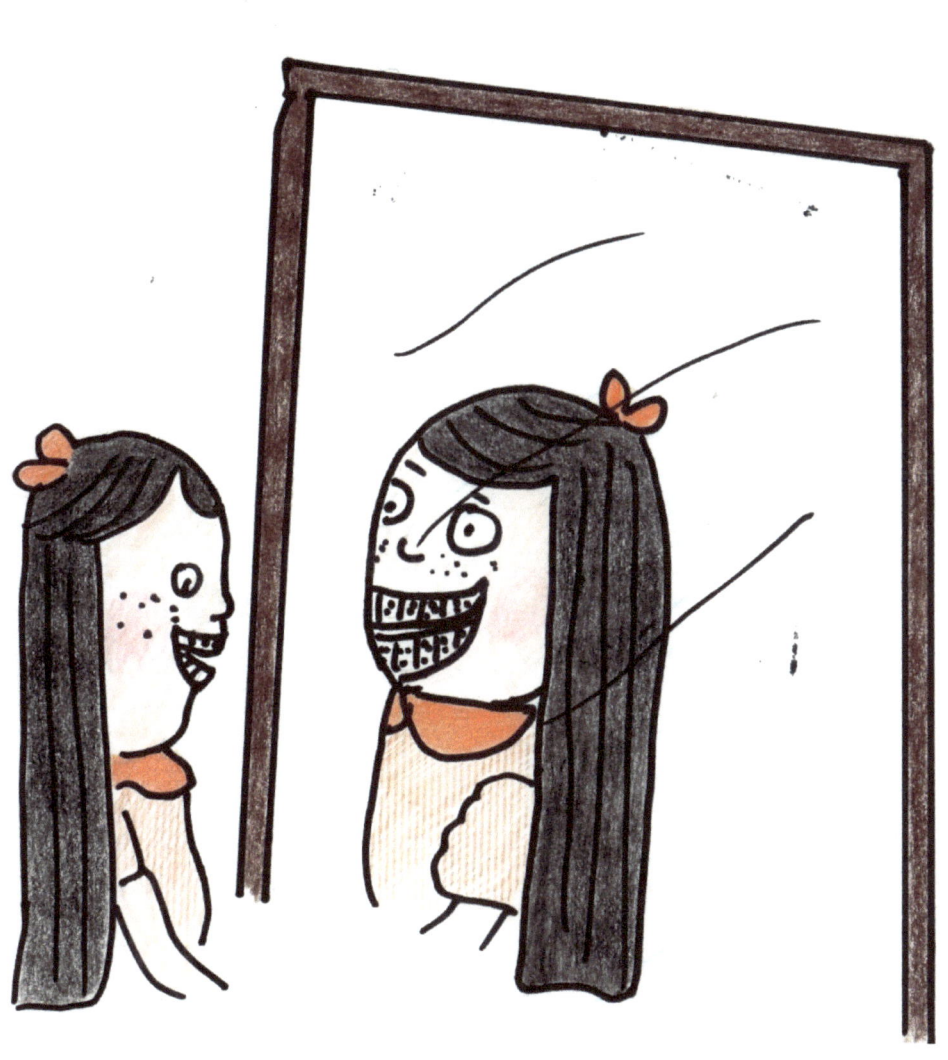

Inside her mouth were some very unhappy teeth.

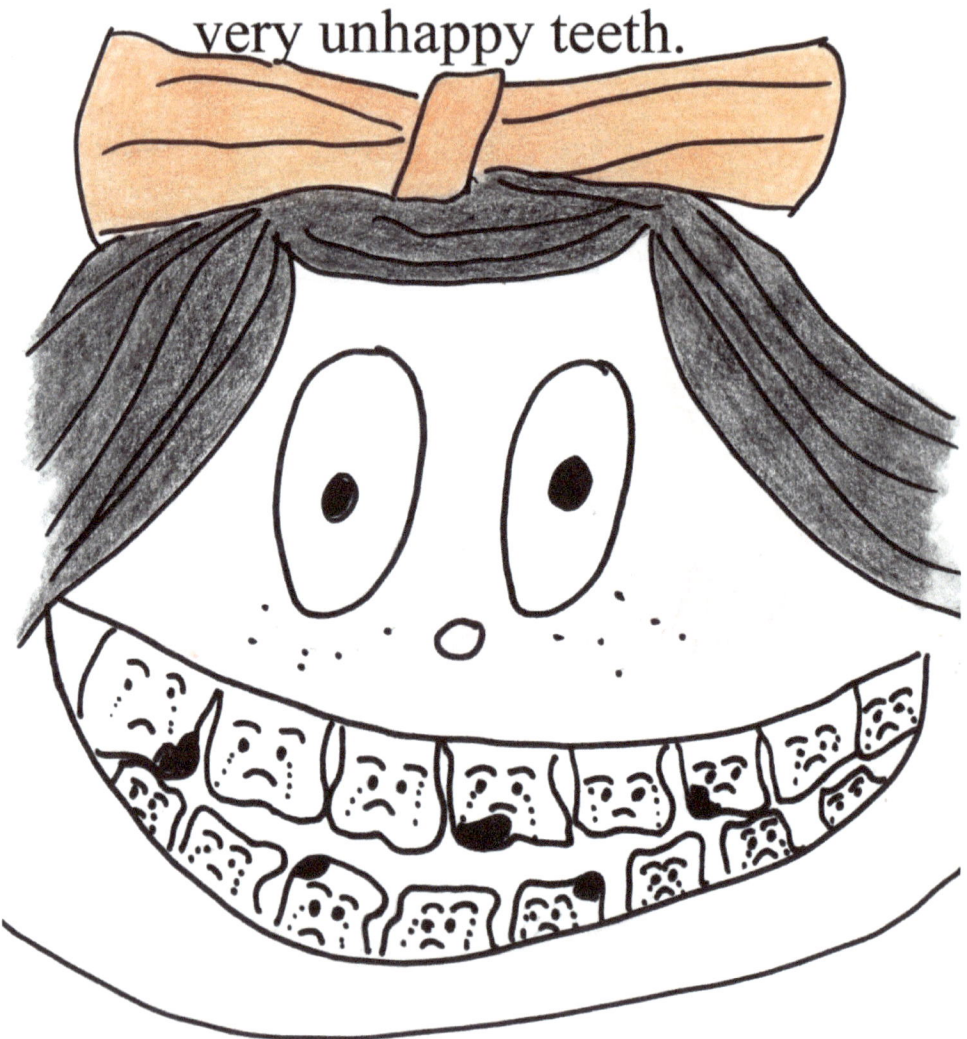

Her teeth said, "You have been eating too much candy! You have been eating too much cake! You have been eating too many sweets!"

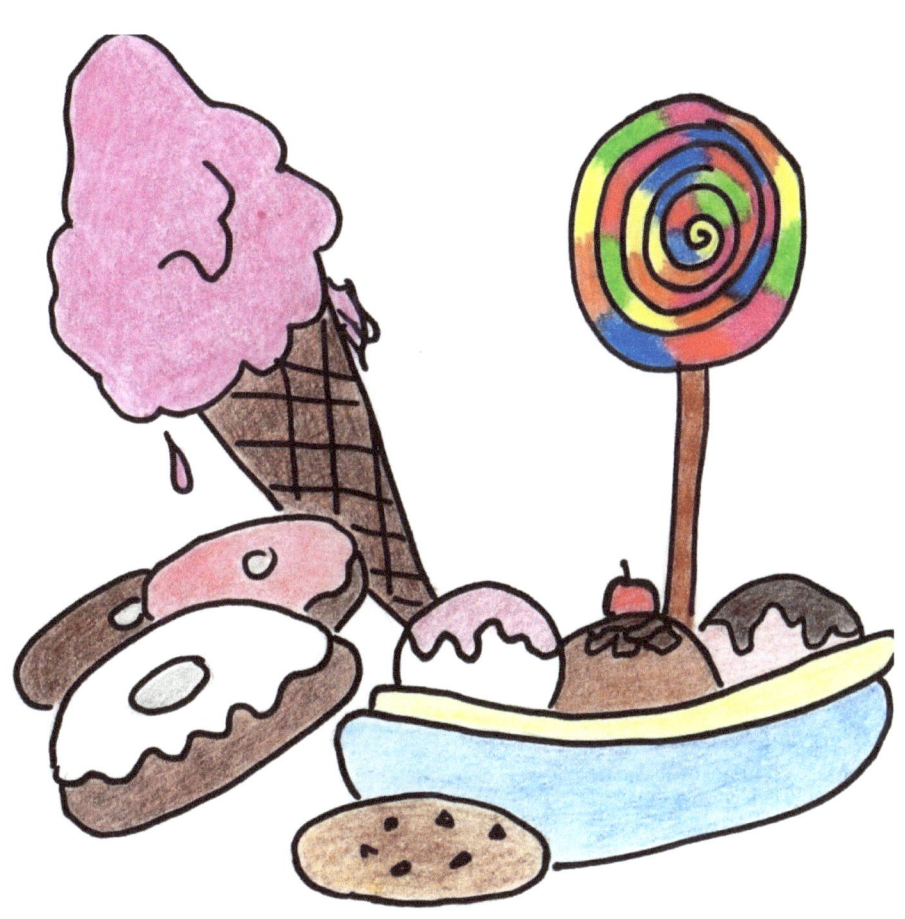

With tears in their eyes they said, "Cavity bugs have eaten big holes in us!"

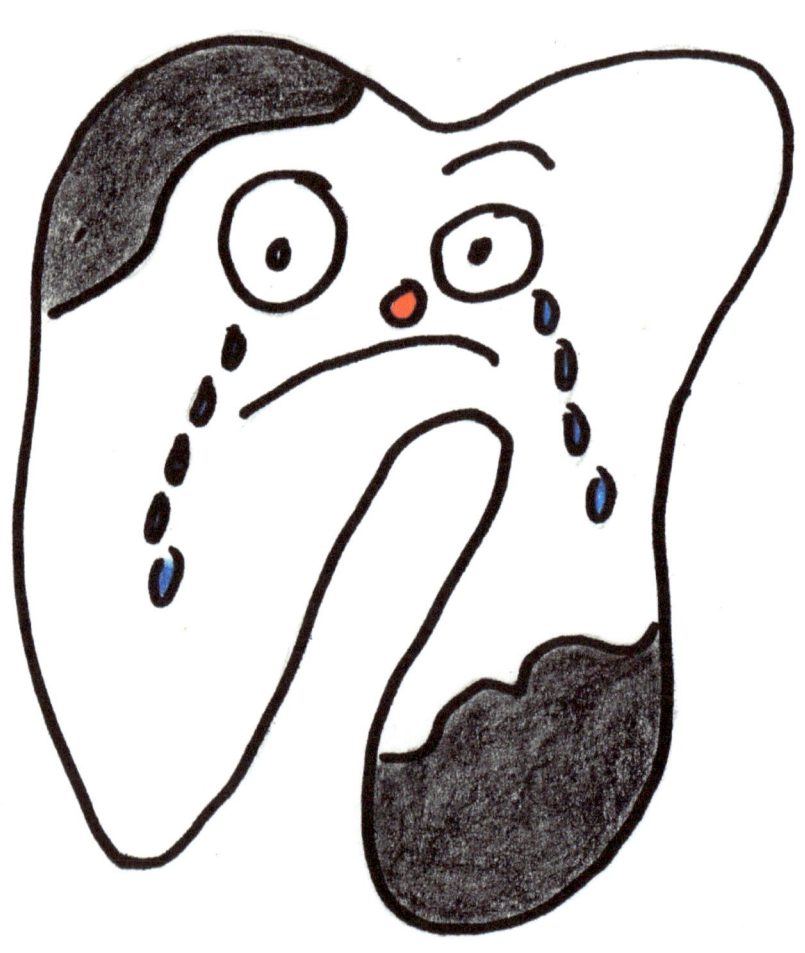

Right away the little girl went to find
Mr. Toothpaste, Mrs. Toothbrush,
And their daughter Flossy.

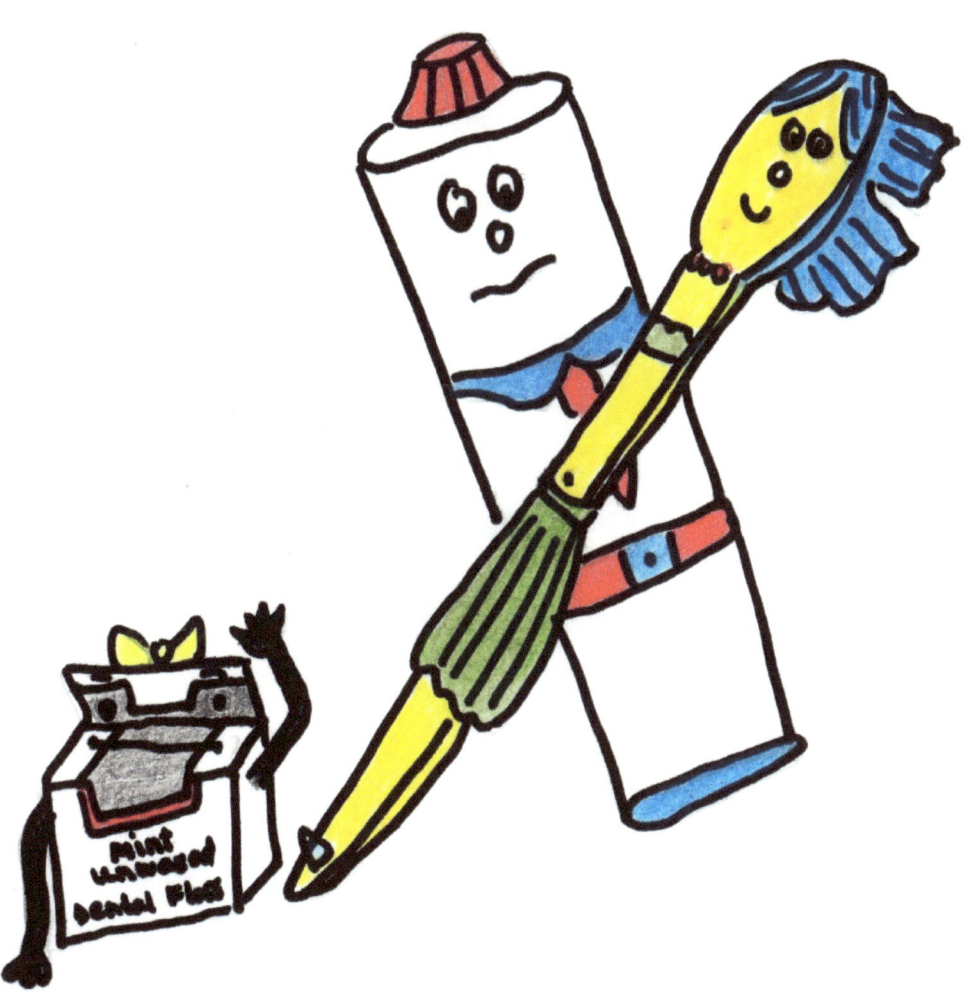

Mrs. Toothbrush said,
"My bristles are soft,
So brush away.
I won't hurt your gums
And I fight tooth decay."

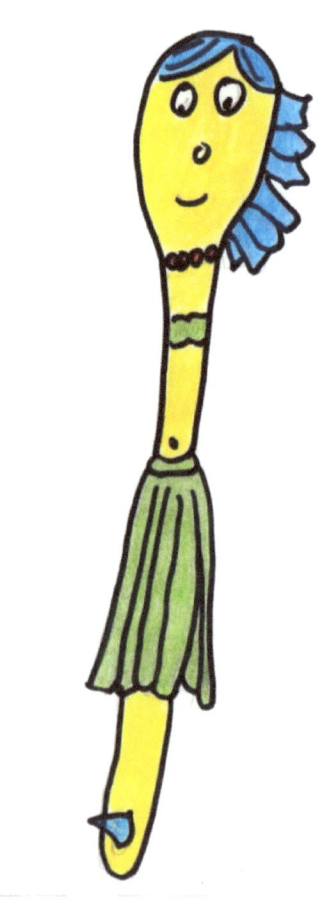

Mr. Toothpaste said,
"I am a big help.
There is fluoride in me.
If you brush twice a day
I will fight cavities."

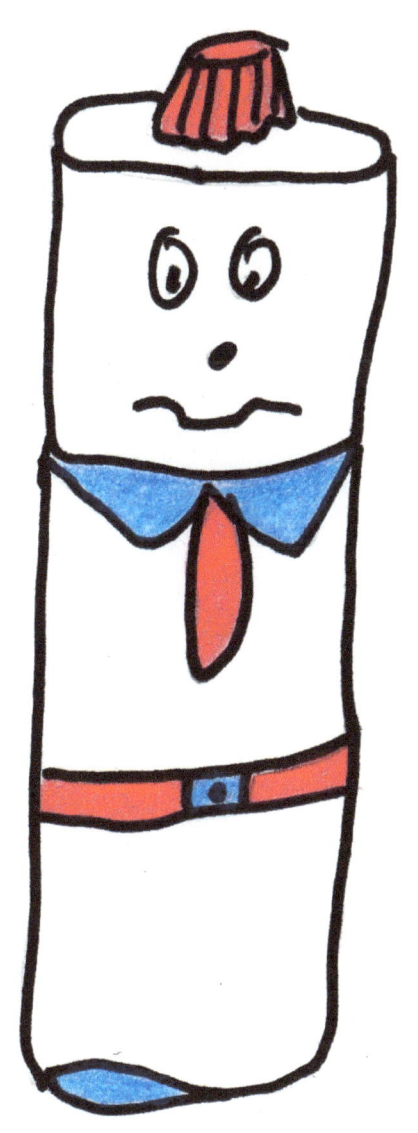

"Hey, what about me?"
Said little Flossy.
"I get out the food that's stuck
In-between your teeth!"

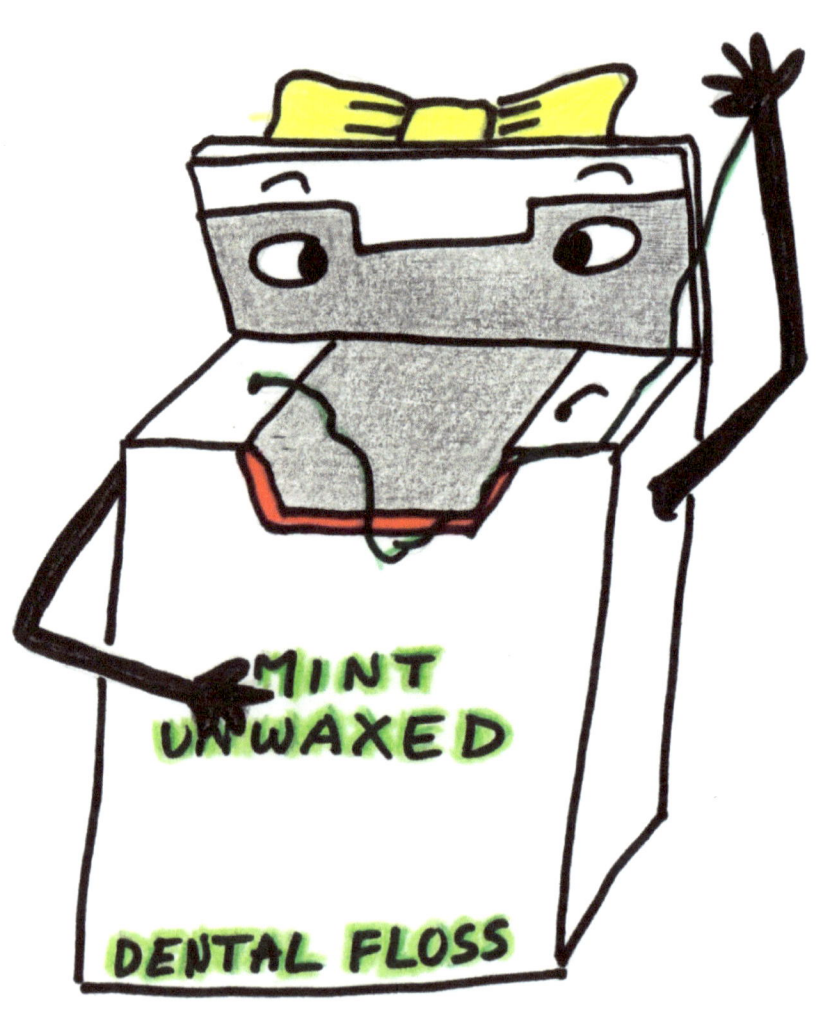

"We work as a team
To keep your teeth clean.
But if you have cavity
Bugs we will scream!
For we cannot help you.
Not a thing we can do.
I guess that a dentist you'll
Need to go to."

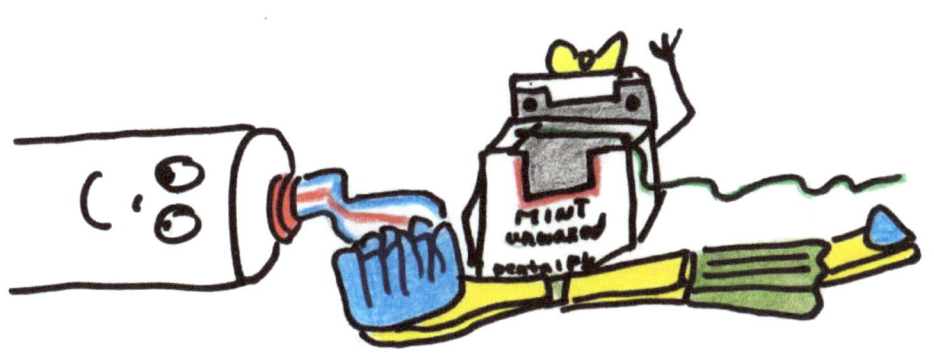

The little girl went to see her dentist.
He chased away all the cavity bugs.

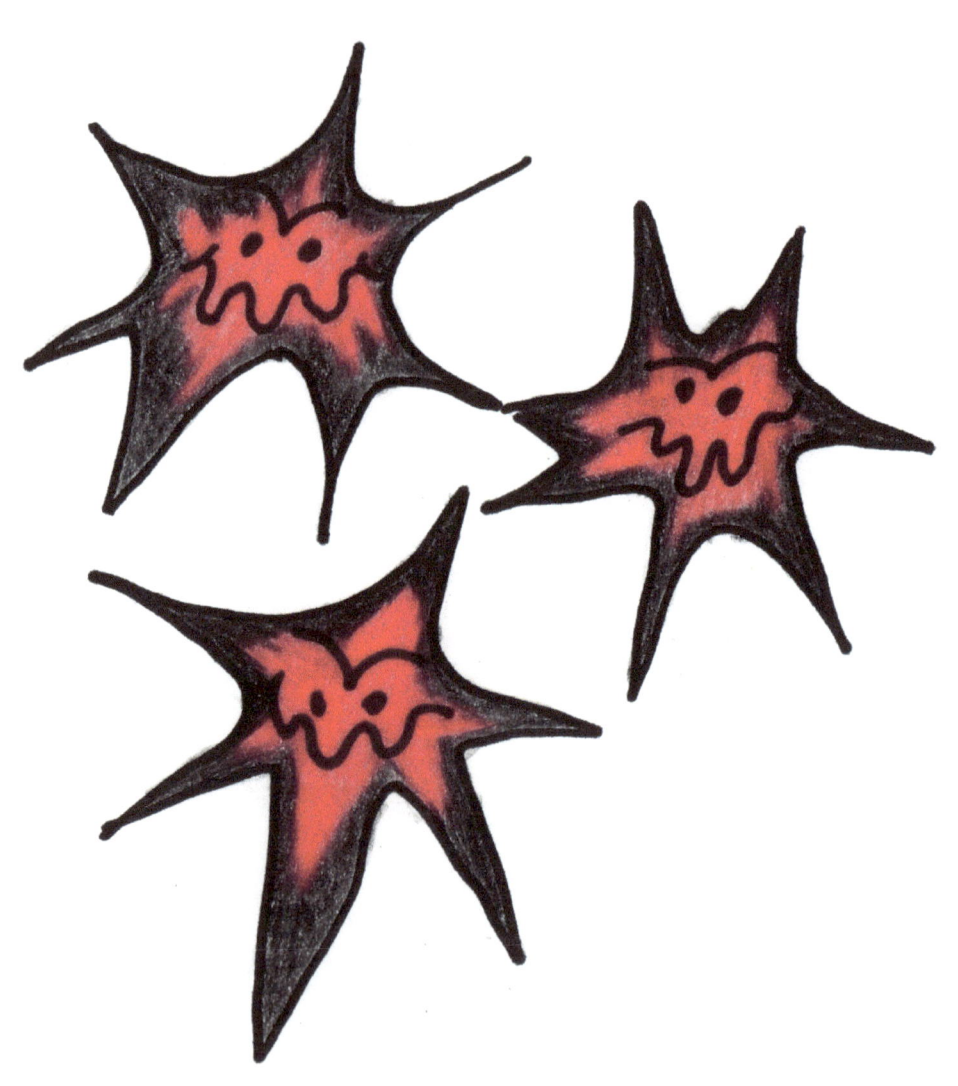

The cavity bugs did not come
back
because........

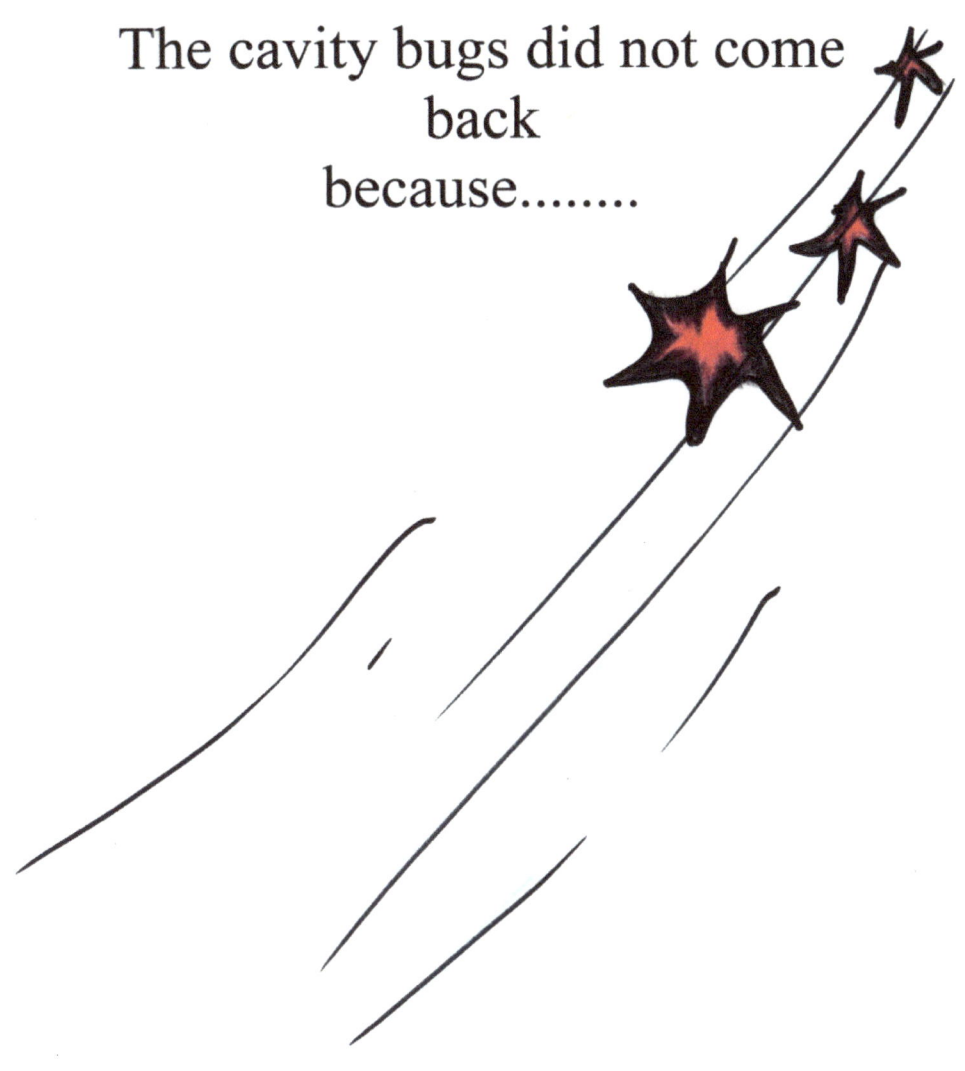

The little girl ate good things
for breakfast.

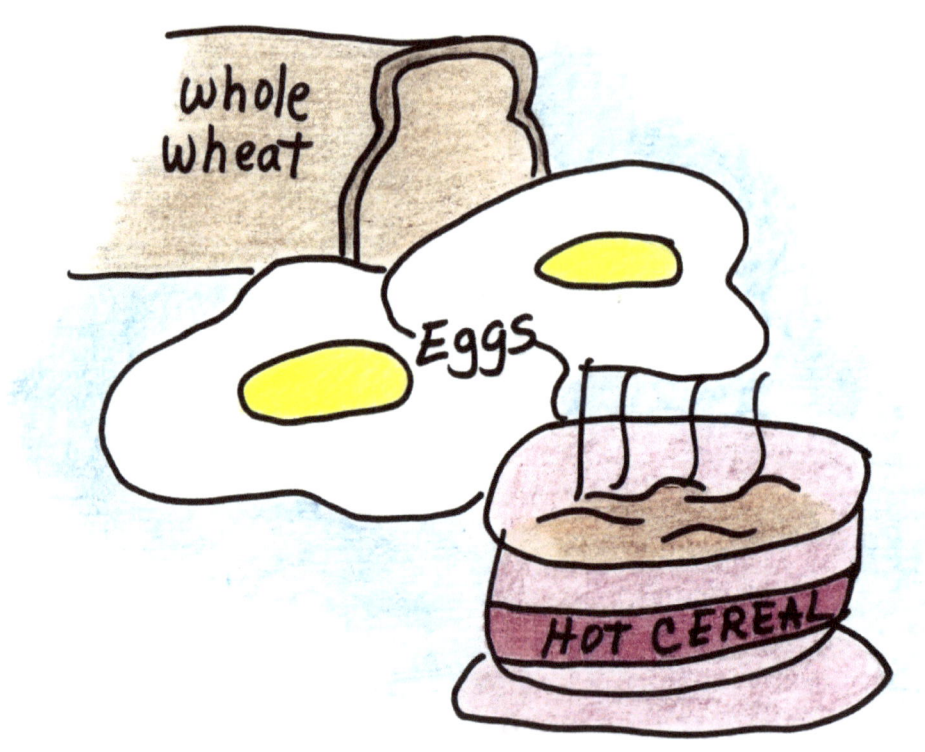

She ate good, healthy snacks.

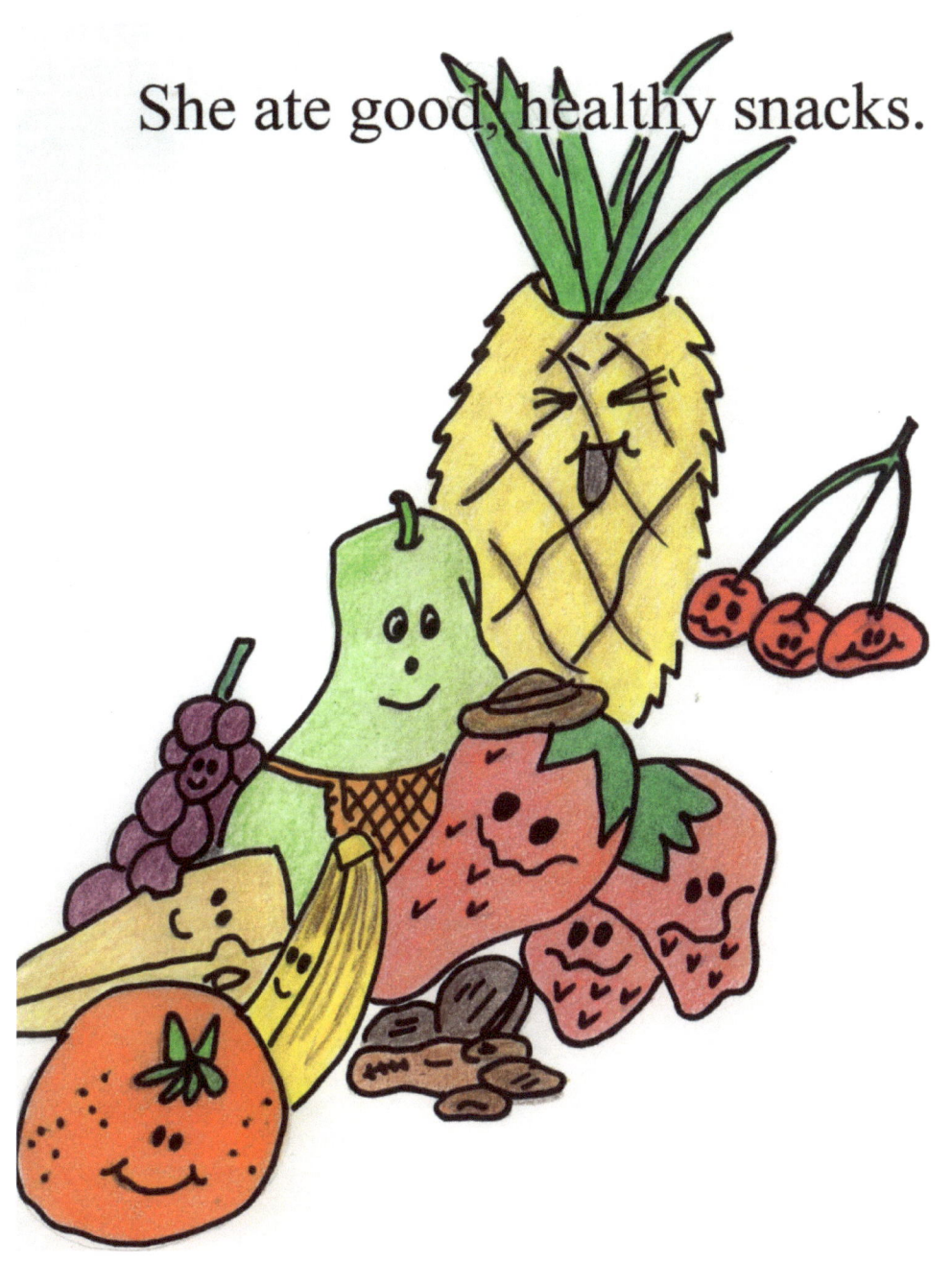

She had only milk at bedtime.

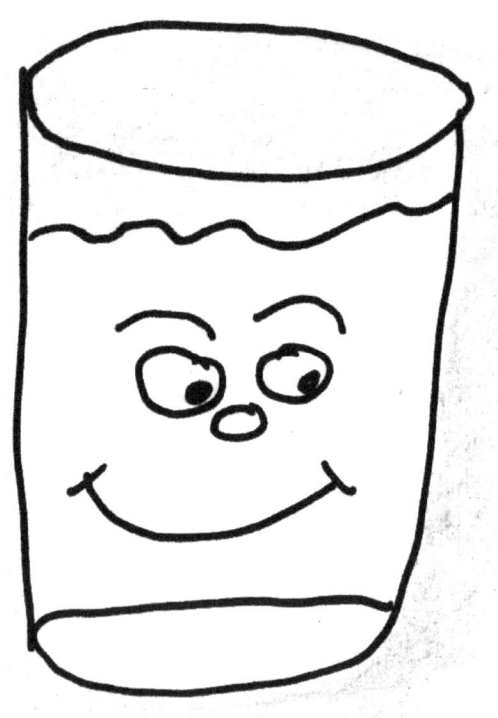

She brushed her teeth in the
morning and every night.
She used Flossy every day.

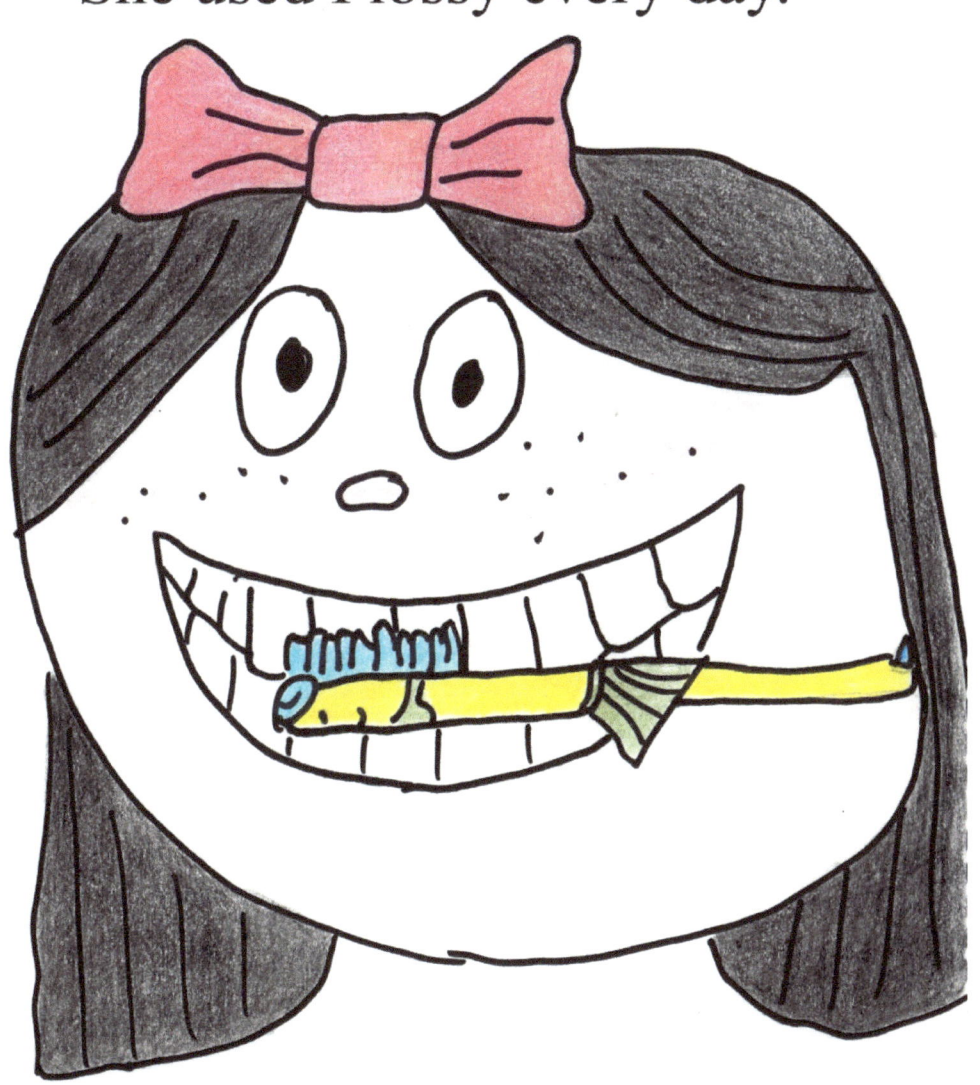

And her teeth lived happily
Ever after.

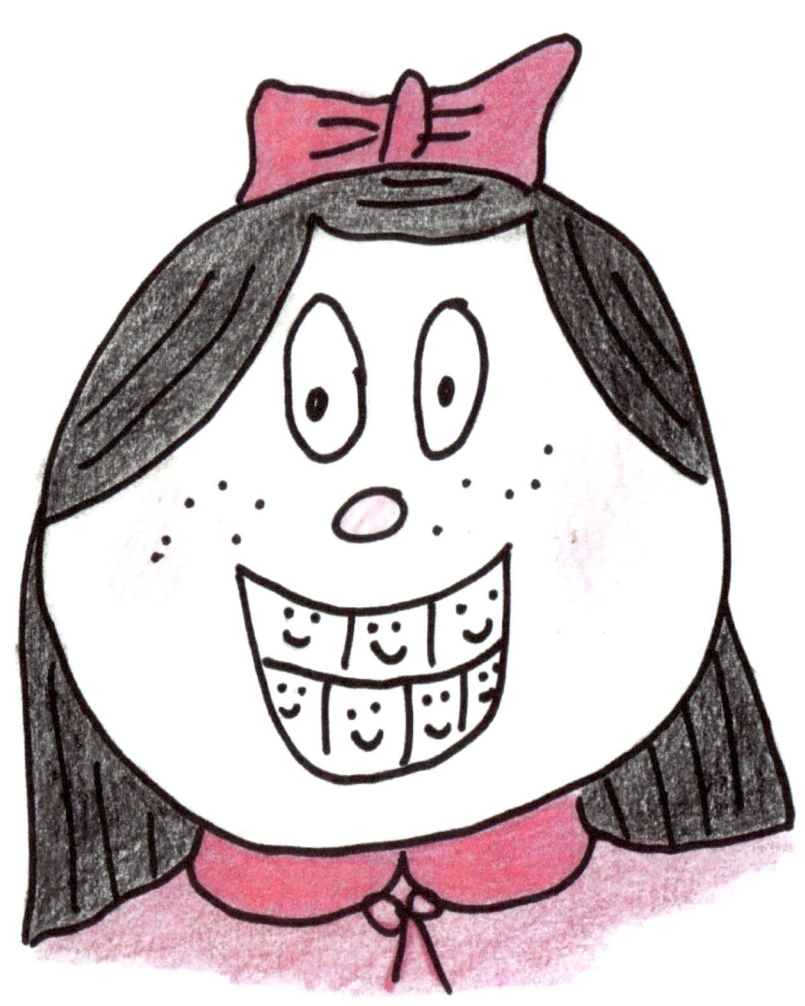

THE

END